SUICIDE... WHY?

Help Me Understand

Bobbie Renfro

ISBN: 978-0-578-34309-9 (paperback)
ISBN: 978-0-578-34310-5 (eBook)

Dedication

I dedicate this book to my family and friends who suffered so much pain they felt suicide was all there was left. I lived that pain, and I am sorry for all your affliction and sorrow.

Gone but never forgotten.

Ed
Chanelle
CJ
Cory
Rusty
Troy

Acknowledgements

I want to thank my husband for being so supportive as I struggled to write this book. I will forever be thankful for your patience and encouragement.

I also want to thank my editor. I am grateful for the advice and suggestions offered, which improved the message I wanted to share with others.

Table of Contents

Introduction

Suicide … a topic not easy to discuss, but everyone wants to understand. "Why did they choose to take their life?" That is a tough question to answer, and even if you can, that answer may not ease your pain.

Suicide results in sorrow, shock, anger, and fear. Fear keeps society from talking about suicide, perpetuating the problem. And talking about suicide *is* important. We face an increasing number of suicides in our society, of both adults and teenagers. When it happens, people are at a loss: they don't understand how someone can take their own life. I want to change that.

The big questions asked after a suicide are often about how and why.

➤ What was so horrible about their life?

➤ Why would they even consider suicide?

➤ How could they choose to take their life?

Other questions follow as shock turns into anger.

➤ Why didn't they reach out for help?

➤ How could they be so selfish?

➤ How could they leave their family? Me?

These questions are reactive to the shock of suicide, but are even more challenging to answer. You may never know the answers to any of these questions. You may never have one definitive reason "why" a loved one turned to suicide. More than likely, multiple reasons pushed them to a suicidal point. I know they did for me.

I attempted suicide, and by God's grace, I am alive. I experienced the psychosis and loss of rationalization that comes with suicide. I will never forget that night; it's burned into my memories, where it will stay for the rest of my life. For the longest time, I didn't want anyone to know, because I was ashamed of what I'd done. I never talked about that night for fear of judgment.

After years of silence, I realized I am not the only one who has thought about or attempted suicide. I needed help, and everyone who experiences suicidal thoughts needs help. There are thousands of people haunted by the same feelings and thoughts I had that night. I am stepping out from behind the guilt and shame to share my story with you, to help you understand the progression of thoughts that can lead someone to suicide.

I am a survivor, and I want to help you understand how suicidal thoughts and intentions (called "suicidal ideations") push someone to take their life. I hope sharing my personal experience with suicide will help you understand how a suicidal person thinks and feels the moment suicide turns from thoughts into actions.

I will not tell you ten reasons why someone attempts or completes suicide. There are a million reasons why someone might think dying is the only escape from their agony, heartache, and suffering.

Instead, my purpose is to help you understand what happens to your thoughts when suicidal. Understand the broken mind of someone who believes there is no escape from the pain.

Understanding how someone can take their life requires an unfamiliar perspective. I am going to introduce a new way of looking at suicide and show you the perspective created from a suicidal state of mind. All I ask is for you to have an open mind.

I can't take your pain away, though I wish I could. Instead, I want to help ease the guilt, grief, shame, or sorrow you might be experiencing. The pain and suffering from losing a loved one, a friend, or even a stranger to suicide is unbearable. I don't think the pain ever disappears, but it may lessen over time.

My intention is for you to realize how much pain your loved one experienced and then be able to process your loss and have peace in your heart.

I feel for you, and I am genuinely sorry for your loss. I have felt that same sadness after losing family and friends to suicide. I also know first-hand what your loved one went through, and thus have experienced both sides of suicide. It breaks my heart every time I hear about another suicide, because I know exactly how much that person hurt, and how badly those left alive will hurt.

I pray for your peace, strength, and healing through your experience with suicide. Through this book, I intend to help you gain some insight into what your loved one went through. I hope this increases your compassion, understanding, and forgiveness if that is what you need.

CHAPTER 1

Why Talk About It?

Some people don't want to talk about suicide because death is frightening. Grasping the concept of how someone can take their own life is difficult, and it requires both knowledge and understanding.

However, when we don't talk about something—regardless of what that "something" is—we cannot spread awareness and knowledge about it. The fear surrounding the word "suicide" immediately stops people from discussing it, so we face an increasing difficulty in even spreading awareness about suicide, let alone sharing knowledge about it. Without knowledge, we cannot learn how to help, and there can be no solution.

Avoiding the topic of suicide doesn't change the fact that suicide is one of the leading causes of death in America. The truth of the matter is, suicide is no longer a tragedy affecting a small population of society. Suicide rates are increasing every year, and they are only going to get worse.

WHAT THE STATISTICS SHOW

> Suicide is the 2nd leading cause of death affecting people aged 10–34, and the 10th leading cause of death overall in the United States. [1]

> The overall suicide rate in the U.S. has increased by 35% since 1999. [2]

> 90% of people who die by suicide had shown symptoms of a mental health condition, this was discovered through interviews with family, friends, and medical professionals (also known as a psychological autopsy). [1]

> 46% of people who die by suicide had a diagnosed mental health condition. [1]

> Annual prevalence of serious thoughts of suicide, by U.S. demographic group:
>   - 4.8% of all adults
>   - 11.8% of young adults aged 18–25
>   - 18.8% of high school students
>   - 46.8% of LGBTQ high school students [1]

These rising statistics are frightening, and prove a severe problem exists in our culture. We must acknowledge that a problem exists and seriously analyze why suicide rates continue to increase. It is time to spread the facts about suicide and what causes suicidal ideations.

Now, for most people, talking about suicide is an extremely uncomfortable process—and that is okay. It's perfectly understandable for the topic to be a discomforting one. On its own, death is a difficult subject to grasp; death caused by self-infliction is incomprehensible.

What is important is that it does still get discussed, despite the discomfort we feel. It is only through addressing suicide that we can come to understand the factors that influence it.

Hopefully, by being more open about suicide, we can make it less of an uncomfortable topic and continue to spread knowledge and awareness. When knowledge increases, fear of the word "suicide" diminishes, and we become more open to talking about it. And talking about suicide is a key factor in reducing suicide rates.

PERSPECTIVE

To understand the how and why of suicide, you need to first take a step back and look at it from an unconventional perspective: a perspective that mirrors the same view of one who is suicidal. This perspective consists of living every day consumed with depression and misery. This constant pain forms a negative outlook, resulting in emotional, mental, and physical torment.

Changing one's perspective on suicide is difficult when one hasn't experienced the same type of hopelessness, fear, and despair. Viewing suicide with happy and healthy thoughts can make it difficult to understand how someone can take their life.

Personal views and opinions stem from your experiences and the knowledge you possess on any one topic. The perspective you take influences your ability to understand a suicidal person's outlook.

To better understand how someone could even think about taking their life, we must first accept how a person's thoughts and state of mind influence their decision-making ability when suicidal. Once we understand a suicidal person's state of mind, we are in a better position to help.

You might surprise yourself with your view if you look at the situation with the same perspective as a suicidal person. You may never fully understand why someone took their life, but changing your perspective is a step towards learning.

The stigma surrounding suicide leads people to view suicide as inconceivable. This perspective keeps people from realizing how emotional turmoil, mental torture, and losing hope can push one to suicide.

If you want to understand why a loved one completed suicide, you must put yourself in their shoes. You must use a suicidal point of view instead of your own, rational one.

It is my intention to give you insight into this unfamiliar perspective: the perspective of a person whose thoughts have turned to suicide.

CHAPTER 2

That Dreadful Night

MAY 14, 2010

I replay "that" night over and over in my head like it happened yesterday. I still remember everything. Sometimes, I cry, and the same sadness rushes back. I will never forget that night; no matter what I do, it will remain a part of me for the rest of my life.

I share my experience with you today as a first step to understanding, a glimpse into the mindset of a person who considers taking their own life.

SO MUCH PAIN

I sat on my light green couch and stared at the journal flopped open on the T.V. tray in front of me. I shook my head to clear the fog; I had no clue what to do with myself. My two-year-old son was sleeping in his bed down the hall. While he slept peacefully, I slipped deeper and deeper into my torturous thoughts, and my agony increased.

Unbearable physical pain from my recent back surgery ravaged my body, but the mental pain I was experiencing felt worse. I had destroyed everything in my life. I yearned for relief from the agony, but nothing came to me except more sadness and misery. I wanted the pain to stop, and it didn't matter what I had to do to stop it.

I slumped on the couch. Tears gushed down my face. I felt worthless. I deserved every bit of my pain because I had destroyed my life.

The journal on the tray called to me, and I thought about writing down all the tormenting thoughts that tumbled around in my head. But instead of writing, I fixated on everything I had lost and hated about myself.

I realized that although I had failed myself, failing my family hurt worse. Pain and sorrow shattered my heart. My husband had left. Gone forever ... never to come back. He had abandoned me, along with everyone else. I knew there was absolutely nothing left for me. Everything I had worked for vanished along with my hope, and I would never get it back. Nothing would ever get better; there was no reason for me to live.

Tonight, my pain and misery increased to an insufferable level. My skin prickled like a thousand knives stabbing me. I couldn't determine what hurt more: my heart or my body.

I couldn't cope with it anymore. I despised myself so much. I couldn't even stand living in my skin. Hollowness spread throughout my body as life drained from my soul. I plummeted into a bottomless, dark hole with no way out.

DEEPER INTO DARKNESS

I stood, consumed with misery, gazing out the sliding glass door into the backyard. My physical pain was overwhelming, and loneliness oozed deep in my soul. Desperate to make it go away, I turned to the kitchen, where I kept the medication I had been prescribed for the pain in my back. I hoped the pills would do the trick. They had worked before, so why not on this dark and desolate night?

I walked to the kitchen cabinet, grabbed a pill, and swallowed it. I waited for the relief I longed for.

I shuffled back to the couch, sat down, and stared at the blank page in my journal. My pen met paper. Words flowed from my mind to my fingers so quickly I couldn't get them down fast enough. All my misery, disgust, and anger spewed onto the pages. A wave of tranquility washed over me, and I welcomed the release.

As I continued writing, the negativity inside me crept onto the page, and the words transitioned from anger to a desperate cry for help. By letting my feelings go, I slipped deeper into darkness. That darkness surrounded me, and I couldn't escape the agony.

I jumped up from the couch and returned to the kitchen cabinet for more relief. I trembled as two more pills tumbled into my hand. Tears streamed down my face, soaking my shirt as I threw the pills into my mouth. I waited for the pain to disappear. So far, the pill idea wasn't working.

I stood over my journal and looked at the words etched there so deeply the page had torn. The frightening words revealed my cruel reality, but I wasn't scared. The idea of living felt like fifteen hundred tons crushing me. The desire to die, to escape that weight, consumed my thoughts.

I walked back to the kitchen and pulled the pill bottle from the cabinet. Gazing at the bottle, I knew a few more would soon bring me relief. This time, I filled my hand with pills, closed my eyes, and swallowed each one as fast as I could.

I walked out of the kitchen, oblivious to my surroundings. I spun back around and snatched the pill bottle off the counter. Nothing had happened, so I threw more pills into my mouth. I yearned to lie down and go to sleep—forever. So, I swallowed more pills.

I swayed back and forth in the middle of the kitchen. My wait was over. Finally, no pain!

Wobbling to the couch, I wiped the tears from my cheeks. I fell onto the couch and grabbed my laptop, struggling to open the lid. The screen blurred, and my eyes strained to see the letters on the keyboard. I stared at the screen because I couldn't remember why I had picked up the computer.

I started typing a message to my husband. He was the one person I couldn't bear to live without, and he was gone from my life forever. He had ripped my heart out and stomped the love from it. The pain of abandonment was unbearable. All my strength, desire, and hope were destroyed because I had ruined our relationship.

Pecking at the keys, I told him to check on our son in the morning because I might not wake up; I was going to lie down and go to sleep.

I pushed "send," and minutes later the phone rang. The ringing pierced my ears, but I let it ring: over and over. Finally, it stopped. No one should be calling me right now; I wasn't talking to anyone.

The ringing started again, and I jumped off the couch, cussing at the annoying noise piercing my ears. I wanted to strangle the person on the other end. I yanked the phone off the kitchen counter, cringing at the horrible sound it made. I staggered to the back of the house and tripped while walking through my bedroom door. I fell on my stomach; the phone flew out of my hand and finally stopped ringing.

Excruciating pain seared through my back and down my legs; I couldn't stand up. Sprawled on the floor, I inched to the bed and pulled myself up.

Lying on the bed, I stared at the ceiling. Tears dripped down my cheeks onto the comforter. My mind was blank, and peace and calm flooded my body. Finally, I didn't feel a thing.

I jumped as the obnoxious ringing began again. I poked at the blurred buttons, finally hitting the one to answer. "What?"

"What are you doing?" my husband's voice boomed.

I slurred, "I'm ... going to sleep."

"What do you mean, 'you're going to sleep'?"

"Exactly what I said. I'm going to go to sleep. Sleep ... I want to sleep now."

Bang, Bang, Bang, echoed down the hall.

"Someone is banging on the door," I whispered.

"Open the door, or they will kick it in!"

"Who in the hell is knocking on my door this late?"

"Go answer the door now!"

I pushed away from the bed and wobbled out the bedroom door. I stumbled down the hall, anger boiling with each step. Heat radiated off my face. My legs felt like concrete blocks; I could barely move. But I needed to get to the door to stop the obnoxious pounding.

INTERFERENCE

I staggered to the front door, pissed off, and yanked it open. "What do you want?" I yelled.

A black blur rushed me, grabbed my shoulders, and lifted me off the floor. It carried me to the chair and plopped me down. I sat, stunned, and stared at this uninvited psychopath, trying to figure out what had just happened.

My eyes finally focused and saw the thing that had carried me to the chair. It was a man dressed in black; the intruder was a police officer.

But I didn't care who the guy was. *Why in the hell is he in my house? I don't want him here.*

This gigantic man stood directly in front of me. I stared at him. He kneeled in front of me, his hot, annoying breath skimming my face. "What have you taken tonight?" he calmly asked.

"I don't know," I slurred, my head falling forward.

"Did you drink alcohol?"

I fell back into the chair, shook my head, and blurted, "Nooo!"

The giant man turned and spoke to someone behind him. I looked up, and a man stood looking at the T.V. tray. My heart flipped. *Oh no, he's reading my journal.* I couldn't remember what I'd written. I really didn't care what he read.

I leaned forward in the chair, trying to stand up, but the enormous man trapped me. I fell back into the chair, glaring at the man blocking me from escaping.

"This looks like a suicide note," said a man across the room. "I'm taking this for evidence."

My head jerked up when I heard another man yell from somewhere in the house, "There's a bottle of pills here that's almost empty. The date on it is from a few days ago."

I squirmed to get away from the man in front of me, but it was useless; I was trapped. My eyes lost focus and closed.

11

The officer shook me. "How many pills have you taken?"

"Don't know. Lost count," I whispered.

"Alright, that's enough for me," he said. "I have something for you to drink. Will you drink it, or will I have to force you?"

I drifted off to sleep, so I don't remember answering him.

My eyes flew open. Something smelled horrible. I pulled my head sideways to get away from the stench.

"I need you to drink all of this, now!" a voice boomed in my ear.

Something cold pressed against my lips, forcing them open. My mouth filled with the most disgusting thing I have ever tasted. A man beside me tilted my head back and poured more liquid down my throat. I gagged at the taste of charcoal. My eyes closed, and everything went black as I drifted back to sleep.

THE DUNGEON

Bright lights blinded me. I struggled to keep my heavy eyelids open. I squinted as I stared at the ceiling, confused. *Where am I? What happened? How did I get here?*

A bunch of wires and tubes sprouted from various parts of my body. I stared at them, shocked. I cringed and whipped my head sideways in response to a shrill voice from across the room.

A woman with gentle brown eyes and a huge smile marched towards me. "How are you feeling?" she asked.

I glared at her, wishing I could slap the smile off her face.

"You are in the hospital. Do you remember what happened?"

That's a stupid question. I couldn't remember anything.

"You swallowed a bunch of pills." Her head tilted, inspecting my face. "Fortunately, you got here soon enough for us to pump your stomach. Any longer, and you might not be here right now."

Confusion filled my head, and I stared at her. She paused and looked away before she spoke again. "We have placed you on a seventy-two-hour watch. Once the doctor speaks with you, she will decide if you can go home."

My face burned as my anger ignited. I bit my tongue so that I wouldn't say something I would regret, and ignored everything she said after that.

I glanced around the room and noticed the door was sliding glass, which opened to a large entryway. Standing outside, to the left of the glass door, was a police officer. I watched strangers walk back and forth outside the glass, but no one looking in my direction made eye contact.

I looked away, and then it hit me why they'd put me in this empty white room. *They think I tried to kill myself.*

At first I denied it, thinking they were all stupid. But as I sat in disbelief, fragments of the night before flashed in my head. I remembered most of what had happened and knew that I'd tried to end my life.

I wanted to scream and throw something at the glass door. I despised everyone around me, and I wanted to strangle my husband for calling the police. He had put me in this dungeon. Rage spread through every inch of my body, and I almost exploded.

I wasn't angry because I had ended up in the hospital; I was only angry because I had woken up. How had I managed to screw up such a simple thing? All I needed to do was take some pills and go to sleep. Every part of me knew that ending my life was the best thing to do: not just for me, but for everyone around me. I was nothing but a burden to everyone in my life.

I thought about how I could get out of this horrible place. Sprinting out the door wasn't a smart option. If I tried, all chances of getting released would disappear.

I lay on the hard bed, contemplating my next move to ensure my release. I wasn't stupid, and knew I had to choose my words carefully. I thought about how to make the doctor believe I was okay. I knew if I said the wrong thing, they wouldn't let me go; or, worse, commit me to a mental hospital.

My irritation skyrocketed as another unwelcome woman walked towards me. Her straight, black hair framed an expressionless face that sent a chill down my spine. She creeped me out. I heard the word "psychiatrist" come out of her mouth and tried to shut her out. It didn't work.

"How are you feeling?" she asked.

"I'm fine. Couldn't be better." I spat.

"You're lucky to be alive; you know that?" she scolded.

Lasers shot from my eyes as I blurted, "Oh really." I rolled my eyes and threw my head back on the pillow. Her words were garbage. I was far from lucky! I turned away and blocked out what she said, but also knew I had to play my cards right.

"Do you understand why you are here?" she asked.

"Yes, I think so, but you're wrong. I wasn't trying to kill myself. I only wanted the pain to go away, so I took some pills to feel better."

"Do you feel like you want to hurt yourself again?"

"No, I didn't mean for that to happen. I thought the pills would help with my pain. When can I go home?"

"Well, that depends on you," she said, her eyes piercing mine. "I want to monitor you for a while to ensure you stay safe—if I let you go home, I don't know if you will keep yourself safe."

"I will not do anything." I sighed. "I am fine. I didn't mean for that to happen. I want to go home."

She stared at me, stone-faced, then pivoted and walked out of the room. I lay down and waited.

The doctor returned after what seemed like hours. "I have two conditions for your release. I will release you if someone stays with you at home, and as long as you promise to call 911 if you feel like hurting yourself again."

The corners of my mouth lifted slightly. I looked her straight in the eyes. "Yes, of course I will."

My insides flipped. I congratulated myself, even though it was a blatant lie. Nothing had changed in the way I felt about myself. Pain still consumed me, and I dreaded life.

There was one thing I knew for certain: if I tried again, I wouldn't say a word to anyone. I would do it right and never wake up.

CHAPTER 3

The Myth Behind "The Reason"

WHAT WAS SO AWFUL?

I have often heard the question: "What was so bad about their lives that made them do *that*?" Suicide is very personal, and the mystery behind it makes it extremely hard to understand. We can't see how a person could feel so bad they want to end their life.

So, how do you get to the point of suicide? Well, the main reason is because you lose hope in life. You may not feel loved, or loathe yourself, or it could be something else that destroys all your happiness. In your heart, you know you are worthless, deepening the hate for yourself.

Suicidal ideations don't result from experiencing a few bad days here and there, and there are rarely one or two distinct sources, or "reasons," behind it. The desire to end your life comes when you have endured so much pain you can't handle living with it anymore. The pain is deep-seated, horrendous, and consumes every inch of your body, making it impossible to function.

THE FIRST TIME

Nineteen years old. That's how old I was the first time I thought about ending my life. My thoughts were always passive, and I didn't have a plan to do anything. But many years later, all that changed.

Looking back at my younger years, I remember forming a negative self-image around the age of seven. Pretty early, isn't it? I remember looking in the mirror and seeing a shy, ugly, fat girl, which was far from the truth.

My internal struggle originated when I first believed the lies I formed in my head. These lies caused the distorted thoughts that haunted me as I grew older. I pretended to be happy, but deep inside, I was miserable.

I journaled a lot before I attempted suicide. The intent was to help me sort out my feelings and negative thoughts. The night I attempted suicide started with journaling, and it led to the worst night of my life. I don't journal anymore.

I recently read my old journals and was shocked to see how sad I was, and how far back my desire to die went. It surprised me, because I don't remember my life being the way I described it in the journal entry.

I found this journal entry I wrote in 2005. I didn't attempt suicide until 2010. This entry reveals how long I experienced suicidal thoughts before ever making a plan and following through.

MAY 20, 2005—JOURNAL ENTRY

I am so confused. I am such a 5/20/05
horrible person. I don't understand why. I
can honestly say I hate myself. God I
fucking hate who I am. I just wish I
wasn't here. No more pain, crying, no
more treating people like shit. I'm
such a fucking failure it makes me so
sick. I don't even know what my purpose
is here. I'm so fucking worthless. I ruin
everything. No wonder ██████ ██████
██████████████ I thought I was something
good + I'm not. No one deserves my
coldness. I'm such a cold person.
What has happened to me? Why am
I still here? I hate who I am
I hate who I am! I hate what
I'm not. I'm such a let down to
myself + everyone in my life.
I'm unhappy so I don't want
anyone else to be. That's not
right. What is wrong with me?
Why am I so negative? No one
will love who I am because
I'm a fucking worthless piece
of crap that just doesn't need
to be here - Why am I
here?

The unhappiness I felt for over five years percolated, resulting in toxic thoughts that distorted the way I looked at everything in life. I never told a soul about how I felt, or that I thought about suicide. I hid it from everyone because I was afraid of their judgment; I didn't need to invite their negative opinions of me and make me feel even worse about my life.

I searched for years to find the next thing to make me whole, but I always came up empty-handed. My happiness lay on the surface, not in my heart.

Over time, my pain piled up, and coping became impossible. I didn't know how to handle my emotions, especially the negative ones, so I stuffed them inside for years. I became a pro at hiding my feelings, and the inner battle I fought carried me down a path where I lost myself.

I finally hit rock bottom. I couldn't handle the pain or deal with my emotions, and I saw no way to escape the hurt except to end my life.

You must realize: once you have endured all the pain you can handle, you believe there is nothing left to live for. I didn't see another way to make it stop. My thoughts were so toxic that I knew, in my heart, that ending my life was the best thing to do.

AFTERWARDS ... DID IT GET BETTER?

When I woke up the next morning after my suicide attempt, dread flowed through my veins. The addition of humiliation and guilt caused me yet more pain. Every inch of my body hurt worse than it had the night before. I wanted to rip my heart out and stomp on it to empty it of the horrible feelings. I didn't think life could get any worse, but it had.

The worst night of my life was the night I attempted suicide, but the dread and despair I felt the night before returned with a vengeance. I wanted no more of this horrible, constant pain, and I longed to be numb again. Instead, I was still alive, and that was the last thing I wanted. Attempting suicide had not relieved me of the desire to die.

DREAD

Have you ever felt dread? If you haven't, it may be difficult to understand how it affects you. Dread is defined as the terror or extreme apprehension of something in the future. A fear so extreme, it can make you physically ill and paralyze you.

Dread feels like five hundred pounds weighing you down and suffocating you. You're empty, cold, and dead inside. You loathe every second you're alive, because you know each day will turn out worse than the one before.

How would you feel if you knew your situation would only get worse and never change? How long could you endure the pain you experience as it piles up on top of you?

When you experience constant misery, fear consumes you every day. You are unhappy, and you dread facing another unhappy day. Eventually, your desire to live disappears completely. You feel alone in a battle against yourself and believe that no one can, or even would, help you.

Living with pain and agony every day makes your life awful. You dread continuing to feel your unhappiness, self-hatred, or worthlessness, and want the torment to end. Your thoughts focus on stopping the agony, and you believe the only way is to end your life.

CHAPTER 4

State of Mind Influence

HOW COULD THEY EVEN THINK OF TAKING THEIR LIFE?

This is the inevitable question asked when someone completes suicide. Whether or not you know the person well does not keep the question at bay. Suicide is an act that most people cannot fathom. It is the ultimate of the unknown, and the unknown scares people. Learning how one's state of mind can lead them to suicidal thoughts will help you understand why someone can even think about attempting suicide.

Suicidal thoughts can stem not only from the current events in your life but, more importantly, from how those events affect how you feel. And the way those feelings, in turn, affect you depends on your state of mind.

In this way, your state of mind is integral to how you make decisions, how you view yourself, how you view your life, and how you process everything that happens to you. All these things combined can lead you to the negative thoughts and hopelessness that pushes you to suicide.

So, how exactly does your state of mind lead to suicide? Let me break this down so you can try to comprehend how suicide can even cross a person's mind.

What does "state of mind" mean? Have you ever really thought about what it is and how important it is? Probably not. Why would you?

State of mind consists of your mood, emotions, thoughts, and feelings, and how those, in turn, affect your behavior and decision-making. All these aspects combined determine how you view your world. Whether you see things like the "cup half-empty" or the "cup half-full," your viewpoint will steer you in the directions you take each day and affect the decisions you make, good and bad.

Your state of mind shapes the way you think about yourself. There are both healthy and undesirable states of mind. When your state of mind goes from positive to negative, negative thoughts, emotions, and viewpoints start to affect your actions.

When you are suicidal, positive thoughts you may have had about yourself and your life slowly change—and sadly, disappear. You may see yourself as worthless, and/or as a burden to everyone around you. You may believe that you are a failure in all aspects of your life, or that there is no conceivable way anyone could like you. If anyone tells you they care, you believe it to be a lie, and nothing can change your mind.

23

Since this mindset is so damaging to your self-worth, it adds to all the other pain you experience. The increase in pain raises your levels of negativity. In turn, your feelings of worthlessness increase to new, heightened levels, and you see yourself as a significant burden to everyone.

It is a vicious spiral, from which hate often emerges. This hatred is not for anyone around you, but for yourself: for who you are, and what you have become. You hate that you even exist.

Self-hatred is only one aspect that can affect your state of mind. No matter what the origins are, this shift in your state of mind manifests in the way you make decisions. The way you handle stress, anxiety, fear, agony, and many other things change. In this state of mind, there is no such thing as a "positive outlook" on anything. At this point, your world dims, and it can be impossible to turn the light back on without help.

Your state of mind affects the decisions you make. Good decisions result from a positive outlook, one where you are still filled with hope for the future. Bad decisions result when negativity is the basis of your life's input.

As the pain in your life increases, your thought patterns change due to the negativity you endure every day. The positive mindset you once had succumbs to constant negativity, and you become blind to anything positive in your life.

When your thoughts are consistently negative, and you remain in that cycle of negativity, you lose the capability to make positive decisions. This toxicity leads to harmful actions, and your pain increases yet again.

The negativity takes over your life and everything in it; your hope diminishes, and the loss of self-worth elevates to damaging levels. You start believing that this is how it's always going to be: that it will never change.

Your distorted perspective poisons your thoughts and destroys your hope entirely, leading you to believe that all hope is lost forever.

Toxic thoughts increase the negativity in your life by continually feeding your thoughts with lies. As you fill your mind with lies about yourself, the lies will eventually turn into beliefs. Beliefs are opinions you learn and trust, but they aren't based on fact. When your beliefs are lies, they drive your emotions negatively and take control of your thoughts and behavior.

COGNITIVE DISTORTIONS

What are cognitive distortions, and what do they have to do with suicide? Cognitive distortions are biased ways of thinking about yourself and the world around you. They are specific ways that you can distort your thinking. These irrational thoughts and beliefs can lead to problematic emotional states and behavior. [3] The only purpose for cognitive distortions is to make you feel bad about yourself.

Cognitive distortions include two main types of thought patterns: misrepresented thoughts and deformed

25

thinking. Both thought patterns cause disbelief in who you are, and result in the inability to deal with negative emotions.

To misrepresent something means to incorrectly, improperly, or falsely present information in a deceiving way. Misrepresented thoughts destroy your self-worth. They are inaccurate, negative ideas you formulate about yourself, which leads to cognitive distortions. As you constantly feed your mind with lies, you convince yourself they are true, not realizing what is happening to you.

Another type of cognitive distortion is deformed thinking. You might ask, "How can a thought be deformed?" We usually think of deformed things as being something physical that we can see. But deformation is anything that is distorted, warped, or misshapen. Surprisingly, deformed can also mean hateful or offensive. [4]

The longer your thoughts remain misrepresented and deformed, the more they change the way you perceive yourself. Your thoughts become twisted, causing self-hatred and the belief that everyone around you dislikes you as well. You believe all the lies, whether or not they are true. As these deformed thoughts intensify, cognitive distortions increase, and suicidal ideations develop.

Everyone has cognitive distortions. However, distortions are quite different for everyone, and each person handles them differently. Cognitive distortions form to help you cope with troublesome life events. Your environment plays a significant role in how those distortions affect you and how you react to your experiences.

When distortions become frequent or intense, problems such as depression and anxiety can appear. In turn, these problems increase cognitive distortions, causing your thoughts to become destructive.

Cognitive distortions cause problems when they become the primary influence on your decision-making. They cause you to disqualify any positive emotional reasoning, even though answers exist. You focus on the negativity and hopelessness because you believe the horrible ideas circling your head are true. There is nothing to change your mind, because you don't perceive the distortions as irrational or lies.

Along with viewing life as negative and hopeless, cognitive distortions cause an "all or nothing" or "black and white" type of thinking. [3] This creates a kind of tunnel vision that eventually consumes your thoughts. You believe life will never improve, and you can't see past the pain, sorrow, and feelings of worthlessness.

Once these destructive thoughts begin, they continue to get worse if not changed. The only way for them to change is to rewire your thought processes.

Do you believe you can control your thoughts in every situation you encounter? Some would say you can always control your thoughts. In most instances, that may be true—if you have a positive outlook on life. Controlling your thoughts is easy if you have hope, and the desire to improve the situations that are causing problems in your life. But when your thoughts destroy your self-worth, and you can't escape the constant pain, that hope and desire die.

Once your hope disappears, your negative thoughts consume you. And yet this negativity is comfortable, because you are used to living with the negative thoughts and emotions. This mindset kills any ambition you may otherwise have to change your thoughts, and it draws you down a path of destruction. This path is horrifying, because you don't even realize you're losing self-control.

It is impossible to control your thoughts when you are suicidal. As I walked around my house that night, I was oblivious to any thoughts going through my head. I didn't know what I was thinking or doing, so how could I control any of it? When you're suicidal, your thoughts control you, not the other way around. You lose the ability to control your thoughts because your negative emotions cause you to believe the lies of your distorted thoughts.

I couldn't tell myself I might be wrong that night, because the thought never entered my mind. I was hysterical, and I couldn't stop the negative lies spinning in my head. I had screwed up my life. I had lost everything worth living for, and I deserved all that afflicted me.

Please do not think I approve of anything that happened that night. That said, I can't change what happened. I don't believe suicide is ever the answer, but when you are suicidal, emotions control your state of mind, not rationalization. Understanding how distorted thoughts change the state of mind of someone who is suicidal is an excellent and relevant start to understanding how you can resort to suicide.

DIFFERENT STATES OF MIND

You now know state of mind consists of your emotions, thoughts, feelings, and how they affect your decision-making. You have a primary state of mind, in which you naturally function, and you experience varying other states of mind depending on your current situation. Normally, you do not experience problems transitioning from one to another. The danger appears when you get stuck in one state of mind and your thoughts become deadly.

Explaining the different states of mind can be confusing, because there are so many opinions on what they are and how many there are. There are three states of mind that are simple to understand. The three states of mind are the reasonable mind, the emotional mind, and the wise mind.

A reasonable mind operates on rules, facts, and reason. When you are in a reasonable state of mind, you think logically and intellectually. This state of mind focuses on facts and tasks you know you can complete. It involves no values or feelings in your decision-making. The left side of the brain controls the reasonable mind by influencing perception, planning, and analytical thoughts. You might perceive a person who is wholly in this state of mind as cold or distant. [5]

The emotional mind is driven by emotions. When you are in an emotional state of mind, you react to your emotional thoughts; therefore, having negative thoughts results in negative actions. Facts, reason, and logic are not involved in decision-making. The emotional mind uses the right side of your brain, which controls problem solving, and emotions. When your state of mind is emotional, the decisions you make are based on your feelings and controlled by your emotions, and can thus become dangerous. [5]

The optimum state of mind is a wise mind. When you possess a wise mind, you make decisions by using both reason and emotion. When you are in this state of mind, you know when your thoughts are true or false. You see the value in looking at all options before making decisions. The wise mind uses both the right and left sides of the brain, often described as the middle of the road: without extremes. Most of the time, you are in a wise state of mind, with some deviation from either the reasonable or emotional mind. [5]

When suicidal, your emotional state of mind traps you, making it difficult to think logically or rationally. Distorted thoughts you believe to be true control your decisions and actions.

My state of mind was purely emotional that night. I thought I'd lost the person I loved the most in my life. I knew for a fact he was never coming back. I acted on fear because that is what controlled my mind.

When you experience an emotional state of mind that consists of only negative emotions and thoughts, you can only fixate on how to stop the unbearable pain devouring you.

IDEATIONS

These negative thoughts influencing your state of mind are called suicidal ideations. Suicidal ideations are not only intense ideas about wanting to end your life, but are also the full intention of going through with these ideas.

When in a suicidal state of mind, suicidal ideations constantly consume your mind every day, and you visualize the plan you have formulated. Rather than fearing your thoughts, they relieve you, because now you know the pain can finally go away.

Let me make one thing clear: just because you have suicidal ideations does not mean you wish to die. The only thing you wish is for the pain to go away—by whatever means you believe will take it away.

There are two types of suicidal ideations: passive and active. Passive ideations are thoughts about dying, but without a plan to carry out the act. Active ideations involve suicidal thoughts, but also a plan to follow through with them. [6]

Both active and passive ideations derive from cognitive distortions and are frequent and extremely intense. When the ideations increase, passive thoughts transform into active thoughts, in turn leading to suicide.

Suicidal ideations develop from cognitive distortions, which increase the chances of suicide. Mental illness can also lead to distortions and ideations, caused by alterations to chemicals in the brain. The correlation between suicide and mental illness is often overlooked because of a huge misunderstanding about what mental illness is. Until we understand the correlation between mental illness and suicide, suicide rates will continue to increase.

When suicidal, experiencing pain (mental, emotional, and/or physical) every day wears you down emotionally and physically. Your state of mind weakens, transforming passive suicidal thoughts into active suicidal thoughts. The only way to stop the unbearable mental torture becomes clear: end your life.

When you continue to believe you cause pain to those around you, the pain, guilt, and shame intensify. The pain I am talking about is not a little hurt from something upsetting, which heals over time, goes away, and then you move on. This pain is incredibly harsh: it cuts deep into the soul and eats you alive. It feels like shoving a knife into your stomach, twisting, and digging it deeper, increasing the pain to unimaginable levels. The longer the knife remains in your stomach, the more the pain intensifies, until you can't go on. Handling everyday tasks and making decisions become inconceivable. The decisions you do make are hurtful to yourself, your family, and your friends; at least, that's what you believe.

As each day passes, your negative perception of life spirals downwards and seeps into your soul, causing the worthlessness you feel to escalate. The pain you constantly experience piles up until you reach the maximum limit of suffering you can endure.

Once you have reached the point of no return, suicide looks like the best option to make your pain go away. You lose the ability to deal with any of your emotions. You don't want to feel them, either, because they torment you when you think about them. This is when suicide turns into your answer, and you give up the fight to stay alive.

Suicidal thoughts can haunt you for any length of time before you act on them. When first starting to think about suicide, thoughts flicker through your mind but disappear, and your pain stays bearable. You're able to function every day because there is a glimmer of hope alive inside you.

However, as the days progress, your pain continues to increase, and your anguish and desperation consume you. You expect the worst out of life, and you plunge deeper into a black hole that is impossible to escape. As your despair turns into dread, suicidal thoughts move from passive into active and turn deadly.

As suicidal thoughts intensify, your depression heightens, blinding you to all things in your surroundings. You sink into a vast, dark hole at lightning speed, horrified you will never hit bottom or crawl out the top. By now, you have lost yourself, and the scariest part is you can't control any of it.

Darkness swallows you, and your mind starts to operate from your subconscious instead of your conscious, pushing you into a suicidal trance or a state of delirium.

Consciousness defines your thoughts, actions, and awareness. It is the state your mind uses daily. Your subconscious is a part of your mind that regulates actions and reactions, but is not currently in your focal awareness.

The subconscious is where desires, motivations, and fear reside, and they can influence what you do or don't do. [7]

When your subconscious is in control, you are not asleep, but you're also not aware of your actions or behavior; awareness doesn't exist. Not having control of your thoughts, actions, and behavior makes it impossible to stop the destructive path you're walking down.

Picture wearing blacked-out goggles and noise-canceling earplugs. You can't see or hear anything, because you are truly oblivious. You long for the pain to stop, and you believe no one will help you, so you don't even ask. The trance you drift into beckons you to end your life. You succumb to your feelings and thoughts, because you can no longer control your insight or sense of reality.

Negative thoughts and cognitive distortions cause most of your dreadful feelings. They negatively affect your mindset, and you become stuck in an emotional state of mind. This leads to poor decisions and actions, which in turn make you feel worse. And the negative cycle continues until your state of mind leads to suicidal thoughts.

Everything begins and ends in your mind. The way you think, what you think, and where your thoughts are focused directs your decisions and behaviors. When you are suicidal, every waking moment focuses on the never-ending, excruciating pain you experience every day.

When you hurt all the time, stopping that hurt becomes your most important goal. The question is no longer, "What can I do to make this pain more bearable?"

The question becomes, "What can I do to escape this pain for good?" The overwhelming misery piles up every day, one layer on top of another, until all you want is to escape it. Your decisions are not about how you are going to live your life; they are now about how you are going to escape it.

These harmful thoughts about yourself are difficult to accept and equally challenging to process. The distortions in your thoughts have changed the way you think for the worse.

What you think is a life-ending problem when suicidal may seem like a solvable problem to one who isn't. The pain you feel is so brutal that even getting out of bed becomes impossible. The pain is complex, confusing, and so strong you want to disappear forever.

CHAPTER 5

Choice or Not

WHY WOULD THEY CHOOSE SUICIDE?

Why *would* you choose suicide? That's a tough question to answer, isn't it? But the true question we should ask is: when you are suicidal, do you even believe you have a choice?

Now, it's important to note that the question is not whether a person in a healthy, balanced mindset acting from a wise state of mind believes there is a choice; it is whether a suicidal person in a negative mindset, acting from an emotional state of mind, believes they have a choice.

When you hear about someone completing suicide without knowing them, you may see suicide as a choice they made because you don't have a relationship with that person. It's even possible you knew that person and still think they had a choice. The betrayal and anger you feel can cause you to believe they chose to die over living.

Personally, I have found that the biggest influence in defining one's opinion on whether suicide is a choice originates from a personal experience with suicide. Without that personal experience, it can be difficult to understand the meaning of "choice" for someone who is suicidal.

The perception you hold about choice results from your life experiences, current situations, and your state of mind. What happens to you in life dictates how you view the meaning of choice. Take a moment and think about the questions below before you move on. How would you answer them?

> ➤ What is the first example that comes to your mind when you think of what a choice is?

> ➤ What does "having a choice" mean to you?

> ➤ Are you open to the possibility of questioning the above definitions in order to look at them from a different perspective?

WHAT IS A CHOICE?

The definition society refers to when thinking, "What is a choice?" is often the simple decision of whether you want to do something. This definition assumes that no harsh circumstances exist to sway one's judgment: that you are able to decide of your own free will.

More than one meaning of choice exists, but this definition we apply leaves no room for other perspectives. Choice is the ability to pick something worthy, excellent, or preferred over something that is not wanted or not ideal. Choice, in this sense, refers to the best or better part of something, not whether it's right or wrong.

If we dig a little deeper, choice includes recognizing that other options are available to you; it's an opportunity to analyze an obvious solution before determining what you should do in the situation. If it is truly a choice, you should be able to acknowledge that another solution exists to solve your problem.

Your state of mind also influences what you recognize as a choice. Your mind steers how you act, react, and live your life. When suicidal, you are in an emotional state of mind, acting on emotions formed by distorted thoughts, which results in suicidal ideations. These cognitive distortions you live with hinder you from seeing all the possible answers to your problem, and thus results in unhealthy thoughts.

When suicidal ideations occur, one question consumes your mind: do you continue living in constant, never-ending pain, or do you do something to end the torment forever? This harmful, unstoppable thought plaguing your mind forces you to suicide. This is not a matter of choosing something "preferred" over the other—it is forcefully resolving a problem of two unfavorable options.

The second part of choice is recognizing your options. When suicidal, your mental state prohibits you from realizing that different options exist. Your distorted thoughts have changed your perspective on life; you don't see other solutions to remove the constant misery and pain.

The pain you experience when you are suicidal is intense. Suicide is about escaping that. Knowing you have no purpose to live, you long for freedom … not freedom from life, but freedom from the pain.

Ask yourself these questions:

> ➤ Would you choose to live in constant physical, mental, and/or emotional pain?
> ➤ Would you rather endure torture when there is no reason to do so?

No, you wouldn't. Suicide results from an unhappy life filled with a tremendous amount of pain and suffering, hopelessness, and the inability to cope with problems.

When you continue to live in unbearable situations, you lose hope, faith, and belief in everything. To you, life is simply more pain, and due to your misrepresented thoughts, you *know* it will never be anything else. If you have no desire for life, does that allow any positive thoughts about anything?

When you live in a state of negativity, you have no positive influences. You don't see good options to help you make any kind of decision, especially not beneficial ones.

When your life experiences are satisfying, you're happy. You may have difficulties and challenges, but you are not in a constant state of suffering. Life isn't atrocious and depressing from the time you get out of bed until you lie down at night. You can make healthy decisions and see a positive outlook on life. Your decisions are made from a balanced, wise state of mind. You are capable of looking forward to your future and the fullness of life.

Now, take a step back ... think about removing all happiness and positivity from your life. You exist in a world of negativity, which strips every ounce of hope from your soul. How do you think your perspective on life would change? Not in an encouraging way. Your state of mind would change from wise to emotional. Your decisions would be entirely influenced by your emotions, and the cognitive distortions you live with and lies you tell yourself would prevent you from seeing any other option.

When suicidal, you are incapable of recognizing opportunities, think of options, or make decisions. If you don't see options to solve your problems, there is nothing to choose from. Continuing to live is not an option, because your pain will continue to torment you. Why would you want to live a life filled with dread and pain?

IS IT A FREE CHOICE?

One aspect often overlooked when determining if something is a choice is whether the choice is freely made. A free choice represents one's ability to perform an action selected from at least two available options. These options must put no one in danger or have influence from outside factors or circumstances. [8]

Outside factors and conditions are the primary influencers on your ideas, behaviors, and actions when suicidal.

Your distorted thoughts drive your behavior and actions. Those distorted thoughts form suicidal ideations, which in turn result in danger to yourself. Knowing suicide results from outside influences leading you to danger, can you honestly say suicide is a free choice?

My argument is that suicide is not a choice; it is a false dilemma. A false dilemma is a fallacy that involves presenting two opposing views, options, or outcomes in such a way that it appears as if they are the only possibilities, even though other alternatives exist. [9] A false dilemma is deceptive, because invalid reasoning makes the options appear better than they really are.

Imagine having only these options to choose from: driving your car into a concrete wall or jumping a hundred feet off a cliff into the ocean. You would choose the one resulting in the least amount of pain, right?

If you look at the two options available, neither one is favorable nor desirable. You wouldn't "choose" either of these options if you realized another, healthy solution existed.

This comparison may seem ridiculous to you, but when you are slipping into a suicidal trance, you become oblivious to your situation and any other options that exist. You no longer have control of your thoughts, behavior, and actions. As the trance intensifies, suicide looks like the best answer because you want the pain to stop, and it is the only thing that will end your pain forever. [10]

Suicide is not an option you freely choose, because you do not believe you have a better one available. You want your pain to stop, and you do not see any other options to make it stop when you are suicidal. When you do not see an available option to improve your situation, there is nothing to "choose" from. So, your options comprise of two things: continue living a tormented life filled with pain, or stop the pain you suffer from every day. Not excellent choices, are they?

Being forced to decide between two undesirable options as if they are the only possibilities is not a choice in any situation; it is a false dilemma.

IS SUICIDE REALLY A CHOICE?

Speaking from experience, when you become actively suicidal, you do not see or believe other options or solutions exist. Your healthy perspective on life has disappeared. When thoughts of suicide consume your mind regularly, your focus isn't on the desire to die, but on ending the constant battle with pain. Suicide, unfortunately, becomes the only solution you recognize to solve your problems, knowing that the alternative, living in unending pain, is worse.

Suicidal thoughts overpower your mind, latch on, and never let go. Your thoughts change when you are suicidal, becoming distorted and making it impossible to think reasonably. When your thoughts are lies, and you exist only in an emotional state of mind filled with negativity, how can that allow you to make a good choice about anything?

I hear the comment, "There is always a choice," but that is not true when you are suicidal. In my mind, I did not see myself with any other options on that horrible night. All I saw was continuing to live with unbearable pain for the rest of my life or taking the pain away by going to sleep. I opted for going to sleep over living a life of hell.

Suicide is not a free choice when you are suicidal; it is the only answer you believe exists. You're not choosing to die over other options; you're admitting defeat in a losing battle against suffering and yourself. If you ask someone who attempted suicide if they had a choice, I believe the answer would be no: they did not see themselves as having a choice. I didn't.

CHAPTER 6

Asking For Help

WHY DIDN'T THEY REACH OUT?

There are many reasons you don't ask for help when you're full of suicidal thoughts. Mostly, the answer depends on how you believe you'll be treated if you reveal your thoughts. You are likely to be fearful of how negatively people will treat you, which causes more anguish.

One reason you don't ask for help is because of the negative stigma suicide carries. Society treats suicide as a criminal act; even in our terminology, it is something that a person "commits." This ingrained attitude makes those thinking about suicide keep it a secret. In this case, the mental illness is not what stops you from asking for help, but the fear of how your family, friends, and sometimes doctors will treat you. You're afraid to see pity staring back at you, and don't want the label of "crazy" or "wacko."

After my suicide attempt, I didn't know how to act around anyone or what to say. I couldn't look anyone in the eyes, because I was so ashamed of what I'd done. I faked every smile on my face and pretended nothing was wrong with me. Pulling away from everyone became my solution to the situation.

I denied I had attempted suicide and convinced everyone I didn't need help. I said it would never happen again, but that's not how I felt deep inside. Instead of getting help, I continued down the same destructive path I was already on. I spiraled into a deep, black hole, and I couldn't climb out.

I pretended the entire night was an accident, but I don't know if my family believed what I said. I did so because I believed my family and friends would never see me as the same person I was before the attempt. I didn't want people to look at me with pity or sorrow.

I thought everyone would treat me like some crazy person, requiring supervision 24/7. Even though supervision was vital for my safety, I refused to admit I needed help.

I didn't talk to anyone about my suicide attempt after that night. Everyone was afraid to even bring it up or to say the word "suicide." To this day, I don't talk about it with anyone except one person.

WHO DO YOU ASK?

Asking for help requires the belief that someone cares about you. When you're suicidal, you feel worthless and believe no one loves you. You believe everyone is better off without you around because you cause them pain. You're a burden, and not one person cares or wants to hear your sad story, so why ask for help?

In this case, you don't reach out to anyone because you don't think anyone can or will want to help.

One time when I was extremely suicidal I called a help line. I don't remember if it was before or after the attempt. The person on the other end of the phone was trying to help, of course, but what he said solidified: no one listened. He said, "You don't want to do that." If I didn't want to do it, I wouldn't have called. I hung up on him because he hadn't helped at all. I never asked for help again.

BEING COMMITTED

Hospitalization is also another reason you might not reach out for help. Having suicidal thoughts is the last thing you want anyone to know about, and one reason why is because you believe you could end up in a mental hospital. When you get hospitalized, you are instantly judged by society. Your friends might think you're different and not know what to say to you, resulting in the loss of those relationships.

Being hospitalized could negatively affect you in the future. The questions asked on some forms or documentation you need to complete could disclose hospitalization for mental illness or a suicide attempt. Answering the questions may not be required, but refusing to answer them causes concerns. You aren't supposed to be discriminated against, but it's possible to be treated differently.

Knowing about what could happen if you're hospitalized horrifies you, so you say nothing.

DO YOU EVEN KNOW YOU NEED HELP?

Sometimes asking for help simply does not cross your mind. Suicidal thoughts become part of your regular daily thoughts and seem normal. Your state of mind is so distorted you don't realize how the negative thoughts harm you. The amount of anguish you experience forces you to focus on stopping the pain. If you ask for help, your pain won't stop, but rather be prolonged, and that isn't what you want.

All these reasons kept me from asking for help, but my main reason was because I felt worthless and had lost all hope. I believed there was no reason for me to live. I was consumed with insufferable pain, and I wanted to die. I didn't want anyone to stop me, and that desperation for the pain to stop led me to attempt to take my life.

CHAPTER 7

But Why?

Back to the inevitable question asked after a suicide. Why? That question is hard to answer because more than one exists.

HOW COULD THEY BE SO SELFISH?

You must admit that most of society views suicide as a selfish act. We find it hard to imagine how someone could willingly take their life, and why thinking about their loved ones doesn't stop them.

But wanting to end your life is not about hurting those around you. It's about escaping the continuation of immense pain you experience every day.

Living with pain every day wears you down physically, mentally, and emotionally. You do not want to pass this horrendous pain on to your friends and family, so you hide your thoughts. Other reasons can include feelings of worthlessness, fear of rejection, and shame.

Suicide is not always about wanting to die, but the longing to escape constant despair, hopelessness, and fear. You feel worthless, and you no longer want to be a burden on anyone.

In this section, I want you to challenge yourself to look at what "selfish" and "selfless" mean from the perspective of a suicidal person.

Selfishness is defined as thinking only of yourself. Selflessness is thinking of others before yourself. When you do something because you don't want to hurt someone else, that is not selfish … that is selfless.

To a suicidal person, suicide is a selfless act because you know, for a fact, that you cause destruction and unhappiness to those around you. These may be an example of distorted thoughts, but when they become the only ones you have, the pain is excruciating, and fear consumes you. In your eyes, the problem is you, and you are doing everyone a favor by extinguishing the problem: yourself.

The night I attempted suicide, I believed I was a burden to everyone and no one wanted me around. Losing my loved ones, my sense of self, and all hope became too much to handle. I was filled with so much pain, all my thoughts could do was focus on stopping it. I didn't wake up one day and say, "I want to die today." Every day I thought about how to stop the pain, and when the pain became unbearable, I acted on my desire.

People assume you think clearly and possess the ability to make decisions when you're suicidal. Remember, when in an emotional state of mind, all behavior and thoughts stem from your feelings. When you feel useless and lack hope, you see no point in existing, which increases your desire to stop your pain. No thoughts enter your mind about how ending your life might affect family or friends, because the tunnel vision of suicidal ideations allows for only one focus: eliminating the pain. Your mind is void of everything else.

Everyone experiences physical pain, but not necessarily mental pain. Mental pain isn't fixed immediately with a doctor's visit; it bombards you for a long time. How long? That depends on the help you receive. Since, as we discussed last chapter, it is difficult to reach out for help when suicidal, it could take a lifetime.

Mental pain doesn't feel the same as physical pain, either. It consumes your mind and body, not just your body. Mental pain extinguishes your hope and increases your desire to disappear.

When enduring mental pain, the reasons that might otherwise encourage you to continue suffering every day disappear. Nobody likes to suffer for a short amount of time, so why would you want to drag your suffering out for longer? You wouldn't, especially not when it becomes unendurable.

When you suffer so much physical and mental pain, you automatically believe you transfer pain to everyone around you—and you don't want to hurt the ones you love. You think more about the pain you cause based on the pain you feel. The only way you see to stop the destruction you create is to remove yourself from the picture.

I did not intend to hurt my family and friends when I attempted to take my life. I only wished to escape the torture I endured, and ending it was the only way I saw possible. The accumulation of pain and suffering stole my hope and replaced it with dread and a fear of living. I couldn't live in fear anymore, and I was tired of hurting my friends and family.

THE EASY WAY OUT?

What do you think: is suicide an easy way out? You might even believe suicide is an explicit choice made to take the easy way. Our culture certainly does … and continues to push the myth perpetuating a lie.

When someone completes suicide, people want to know why. When there isn't a straightforward answer, the blame reverts to the one who completed suicide. Instead of being shown compassion, the individual gets blamed by saying it is an "easy way out." Blaming someone validates the anger that others feel after a suicide and makes it easier to accept what happened.

From the outside, suicide appears as an "easy way out." After all, suicide is a reaction to some type of negative situation, unhappiness, or very harsh, painful feelings. People mistakenly assume that a suicidal person sees the option of taking their own life, as well as the other options for ending the pain they experience, and still choose suicide. That is not the case.

On average, we don't suffer the constant negativity, cognitive distortions, and emotional, mental, or physical pain that can lead to suicidal ideations. We don't understand that living in a wholly emotional state of mind leads to further worse decisions, and that a suicidal person thus no longer sees the other options that are available.

Why are we so quick to say suicide is an easy way out? The negative stigma and lack of knowledge surrounding suicide are the primary reasons for the deep-rooted, inaccurate ideas. The adverse comments that have been repeated for hundreds of years still influence views on suicide.

The misconception of facts about suicide also perpetuates the disapproval of suicide, and keeps us from increasing our knowledge about it.

You must understand that as pain exceeds your ability to cope day-to-day and suicidal thoughts consume your mind, suicide is not an "easy way." It is the *only* way, in your mind, to end the suffering.

In the end, knowing a specific reason "why" someone resorts to suicide may not ease your grief. Instead of focusing on the why, try to understand the excruciating pain a person experiences when suicidal. Try to find compassion instead of anger to heal your grieving heart.

CHAPTER 8

Mental Illness and Suicide

WHAT IS MENTAL ILLNESS?

Do you know what mental illness is? Does your knowledge consist of information you learned on T.V., through the media, word of mouth, or facts? Not everyone has a solid knowledge base about mental illness, how it affects people, or how those suffering get treated by society.

The lack of knowledge surrounding mental illness is prevalent within our current culture. However, knowing the facts about mental illness and spreading that information becomes important if one wants to understand how mental illness links to suicidal thoughts.

Understanding any kind of mental illness starts with knowing the true meaning of the term, "mental illness," itself. The medical definition of mental illness used by psychologists comes from the DSM-5. The DSM-5 (The Diagnostic and Statistical Manual of Mental Disorders, 5th Edition) is the handbook used by health care professionals in the United States as the authoritative guide to the diagnosis of mental illnesses. The DSM contains descriptions, symptoms, and other criteria for diagnosing mental illness and disorders. [11]

According to the DSM-5, the definition of a mental disorder is a syndrome characterized by a clinically significant disturbance in an individual's cognition, emotional regulation, or behavior that affects their mental functioning. They are usually associated with significant distress or disability in social, occupational, or other important activities. [12]

"Mental disorder" and "mental illness" are terms that are often used interchangeably. You might wonder what the difference between the two is. The difference is minor, and often gets interpreted differently in different situations.

A mental disorder is often described as a disturbance of the mental health of the mind. This disturbance is also referred to as "derangement," and may cause confusion or disarray. [13] Many of these disorders can cause very mild to severe impairment. When impairment occurs, activities in one's life become complicated and unmanageable, leading to the inability to make healthy and rational decisions. [14]

This definition comes from a prior understanding of mental health, when it was thought that a mental disorder affected only the mind. With the advancement in medical research, a more current definition reveals that mental disorders affect the brain, not just the mind, affecting the functioning of an individual on a physical level. [13]

Mental illness, on the other hand, refers to poor health resulting from disease of the mind or body affecting the emotions, thinking, and behaviors of an individual. This definition refers to both mind and body.

One way a mental illness affects the mind through the body is by the alteration of chemicals in the brain. The nervous system contains chemicals that promote the communication between neurons in the brain. When chemicals are altered, one's control of thoughts, behaviors, and actions diminish, causing unstable thoughts. When an imbalance occurs, the ability to form coherent ideas and make good decisions becomes difficult, if not impossible.

Before mental health was better understood, experts believed that the term "disorder" was a better fit than "illness." As mental illness studies expanded, psychologists and scientists found that mental illness is, in fact, a disease of the mind and body, and thus used the term "mental illness" more widely. [13]

Interchanging disorders and illnesses confuse our culture. To ease some of this confusion, we must spread the facts about mental illness and make them more accessible.

HISTORY OF MENTAL ILLNESS

Mental illness was discovered as far back as the Stone Age, but was perceived then as merely abnormal behavior. Behavior that differed from what society expected wasn't acceptable, and those displaying abnormal behavior were often silenced or controlled, because they were thought of as animals and thus a threat to society.

As mental illness became more widely recognized, it was thought of as a disease of the mind caused by sins, demons, brain damage, or gods. Treatments used to cure the diseases started with drilling holes in skulls, exorcisms, and bleeding. As time passed, treatments graduated to lobotomies, shock, and experimental surgeries. [15]

This lack of knowledge on how to treat mental illnesses encouraged doctors to experiment on individuals with these illnesses to find cures for their abnormal behavior. To that end, patients were kept in hospitals or asylums. Unfortunately, many of these facilities turned into dungeons, resulting in the abuse and neglect of the patients.

Three theories about mental illness have developed throughout the centuries, but each period has usually been dominated by a single theory, which determined the treatment patients received. [16] The theories didn't improve throughout history but instead turned cyclical, recurring from century to century. The general theories used were supernatural, somatogenic, and psychogenic.

Supernatural theories proposed the causes to be possession by demonic spirits, curses, angry gods, eclipses, planetary gravitation, and sin. [16]

Somatogenic theories identified disturbances in physical functioning caused by illness, genetics, an imbalance in the brain, or brain damage. [16]

Psychogenic theories focused on traumatic or stressful experiences, incomplete or faulty experiences, or distorted perceptions. [16]

Treatment throughout history wasn't necessarily to help the mentally ill, but to ease the fears society holds about mental illness. Fortunately, treatment of mental illness has improved through the years, moving from brutal treatment to a more compassionate approach.

PROGRESSION OF TREATMENT

The discovery of mental illness occurred as early as 6500 BCE, although no medical term existed to describe abnormal behavior—supernatural theories and treatments were the approach for this period. The first treatment performed on patients included drilling holes in skulls. Some treatments were successful in certain illnesses, resulting in the continuation of this brutal treatment. [17]

Around 400 BCE, Hippocrates (460-370 BCE) theorized that an imbalance in the humors (the blood, yellow bile, black bile, and phlegm) caused physical and mental illness. Hippocrates did not believe mental illness was shameful, and that individuals should be cared for at home. This somatogenic theory dominated the Greek period. [16]

Between the 11th and 15th centuries during the Middle Ages, supernatural theory resurfaced and dominated the treatment of mental illness. For instance, during the 13th century, the mentally ill were accused of being witches, and so began the hunting and burning of these so-called witches.

In the 16th century, the establishment of hospitals and asylums were designed to confine not only the mentally ill but also the homeless, unemployed, and criminals. The idea was to protect society from these dangerous people who couldn't control themselves.

Governments became responsible for providing care, and the infamous hospital St. Mary of Bethlehem, or "Bedlam," formed in London. [18] Treatments in the 16th century became cruel and torturous punishment rather than helping with the mental illness.

The 18th and 19th centuries showed a movement towards moral treatment for the mentally ill. Dorothea Dix was an advocate for improving the standard of care. Instead of treating the mentally ill like animals, compassion started replacing the abuse. [15]

In America, overcrowding and the inability to care for the increase in individuals entering asylums became difficult. Treatment reverted to abuse, and patients in asylums received punishment for their abnormal behavior rather than help to improve it.

State hospitals formed, and treatment of the mentally ill became the responsibility of the state. The theories Hippocrates had established reappeared, and the moral treatment of patients was re-established. The 19th century treatment of mental illness reverted to somatogenic and psychogenic theories.

The 20th century brought a more promising treatment called psychoanalysis, which was considered a psychogenic theory. [16] This theory included using psychotropic medications to treat the chemical imbalances in the brain. Psychoanalysis became a successful treatment for mental illness and the most promising for improving it.

The great strides made in research on mental illness have undoubtedly benefited those who suffer from it. Improvements in research have taught psychotherapists that mental illness is not caused by chemical imbalances in the brain alone, but also life experiences, other social factors, and genetics.

Regardless of the progress in research and treatments produced by doctors, society continues to label patients as outcasts or criminals.

WHY THE NEGATIVE STIGMA?

The stigma of mental illness derived from the original beliefs formed centuries ago about abnormal behavior. Even though the beliefs were incorrect, proper information about mental illness didn't develop until years after mental illness emerged. Doctors didn't know what caused the abnormal behavior, and therefore did not know how to treat what is now called mental illness.

Society feared the mentally ill, because it was thought that the mentally ill were dangerous and couldn't control themselves. The solution became to separate the mentally ill from the rest of society. The inability to help mentally ill individuals resulted in doctors using abuse and neglect to control and punish their patients.

Through the years, the horrible perception about mental illness worsened because society's knowledge never changed. Even though advancement in research proved old beliefs about mental illness had created false ideas, that information failed to reach society and improve their knowledge of the conditions.

Some within society believe mental illness isn't real, and that people only fake having an illness to receive attention. Sadly, our culture also believes individuals with mental illness are disturbed or "not right in the head." This horrible misrepresentation of mental illness is degrading and harmful, because those with a mental illness do not choose to have one.

One aspect even more devastating is the increased discrimination individuals receive if they have a mental illness.

The way movies, media, and society continue to portray mental illness exacerbates the negative view kept by today's culture. The progress in research on mental illness, which is based on facts, is not reflected in how we deal with mental illness or suicide.

To improve the current stigma, we must extinguish the fear of talking about mental illness and suicide. It is possible to change the perspective on mental illness, but we must first change our actions if we expect suicide rates to decrease.

THE LINK BETWEEN MENTAL ILLNESS AND SUICIDE

Studies show an undeniable link between the existence of mental illness and an individual attempting or completing suicide. According to the National Alliance on Mental Illness, 90% of people who die by suicide had shown signs of mental illness, while 46% had been medically diagnosed. Unfortunately, 60% of those individuals do not receive treatment for their mental condition. [19]

Leaving mental illness undiagnosed, untreated, and ignored contributes to suicidal ideations and increases the risk of suicide.

There are two crucial points to keep in mind when linking mental illness and suicide.

(1) If you have a mental illness, it does not mean you will resort to suicide.

(2) When someone completes suicide, it does not mean mental illness was present.

The presence of mental illness is a key correlation to suicide (that is, they are linked to each other), but it is not always the cause.

Mental illness changes your state of mind by negatively influencing your thoughts, emotions, and behavior. As emotional strife increases, your state of mind operates on pure emotion. The shift in your state of mind causes distorted thoughts you can't control, and it affects your ability to make decisions. When your state of mind is emotional, it becomes difficult to analyze your situation, recognize options, or realize your situation can improve. Since your thoughts consist of lies, no decision you attempt to make will produce a positive result.

The night I attempted suicide, I remember walking through my house feeling depressed, disconnected from reality, and hopeless. The only thought that crossed my mind was going to sleep, because I couldn't see anything past stopping the pain. My emotions controlled my thoughts, and going to sleep became my desire until I followed through.

Mental illness may not always be present in every suicide, but it increases the risk of suicidal ideations. Mental illness is difficult to live with and affects you in so many ways, making every day a struggle. When you add pain to the struggle, life becomes miserable. You can only endure so much pain until you break down.

The increase in suicide rates proves a need for awareness of mental illness and of suicide prevention. People need to know how mental illness increases the risk of suicide attempts. Reducing suicide rates requires an increase in knowledge about suicide prevention and mental illness. Spreading knowledge and improving communication about both subjects becomes important if we expect to decrease suicide rates.

A LOOK AT MENTAL ILLNESS STATISTICS

Have you ever looked at the statistics of mental illness? The numbers are shocking, and what's more alarming is these are only the reported cases of individuals with a mental illness. Fear of the negative stigma keeps many people from admitting to mental illness, causing the issue to appear unimportant and not in need of attention. It makes you wonder how many more cases are unreported, resulting in higher numbers than disclosed.

Mental illness affects not only the one suffering, but also the family, community, and the world. Mental illness does not discriminate against anyone's age, sex, ethnicity, or demographics. All people are subject to mental illness.

Look at these statistics, updated in 2021, regarding mental illness.

- ➤ 20.6% of U.S. adults experienced mental illness in 2019 (51.5 million people). This represents 1 in 5 adults. [1]

- ➤ 5.2% of U.S. adults experienced a serious mental illness in 2019 (13.1 million people). This represents 1 in 20 adults. [1]

- ➤ 3.8% of U.S. adults experienced a co-occurring substance use disorder and mental illness in 2019 (9.5 million people). [1]

- ➤ Half of all mental illnesses begin by age fourteen, and three-quarters by age twenty-four. [20]

Mental illness affects teenagers as well, which is noticeable when you see the rising numbers of suicide rates amongst that age group.

> 16.5% of U.S. youth aged 6–17 experienced a mental illness in 2016 (7.7 million people). [1]

> High school students with significant symptoms of depression are more than twice as likely to drop out compared to their peers. [1]

> Students aged 6–17 with mental, emotional, or behavioral concerns are three times more likely to repeat a grade. [1]

> 70.4% of youth in the juvenile justice system have a diagnosed mental illness. [1]

Society tends to ignore what they cannot see, but mental illness has a dramatic effect on communities, nonetheless.

> Mental illness and substance use disorders are involved in 1 out of every 8 emergency department visits for a U.S. adult (estimated 12 million visits). [1]

> Mood disorders are the most common cause of hospitalization for all people in the U.S. under age forty-five (after excluding hospitalization relating to pregnancy and birth). [1]

> 20.5% of people experiencing homelessness in the U.S. have a serious mental health condition. [1]

MENTAL ILLNESS CLASSIFICATIONS

All mental illnesses have a specific classification. There are at least fifteen classifications for mental illnesses. Within each of these classifications, there are anywhere from two to ten disorders that are considered mental illnesses.

Mental illnesses such as bipolar disorder, schizophrenia, or obsessive-compulsive disorder are well-known and currently recognized as mental illnesses.

The most prevalent mental illnesses involved with suicide attempts are depression and substance abuse. Society treats substance abuse as an addiction, and depression as simple sadness that will go away, not mental illnesses. These two disorders often go overlooked without acknowledging the need for professional help.

Depression and substance abuse are only two mental illnesses contributing to the increase in suicide attempts. There are several other afflictions not culturally recognized as mental illnesses listed in the DSM-5.

The chart below lists the disorders classified as mental illnesses, some of which you may not realize are considered a mental illness. [21] The list does not contain all disorders listed in the DSM-5, but the more common conditions recognized by doctors.

MENTAL ILLNESS DISORDERS	
Anxiety Disorders	• Panic Disorder • Anxiety Disorder
Bipolar & Related Disorders	• Depressive Episode • Manie Episode
Depressive Disorders	• Major (Clinical) Depressive Disorder • PMDD (Premenstrual Dysphoric Disorder) • Substance/Medication-Induced Depressive Disorder
Dissociative Disorders	• DID (Identity Disorder- At least two personality states) • Dissociative Amnesia (Unable to remember essential life knowledge)
Disruptive, Impulse Control & Conduct Disorders	• Kleptomania (Inability to resist urges to steal) • Pyromania (Inability to resist impulses to set fires) • IED (Intermittent Explosive-repeated impulsive, violent episodes of anger outbursts)
Eating Disorders	• Anorexia • Bulimia • Binge-eating
Neuro-developmental Disorders	• Autism • ADHD (Attention-deficit) • Intellectual Disability (Below average mental ability and lack of skills for day to day living) • Communication/Speech Disorders
Obsessive-Compulsive Disorders	• OCD (Obsessive Compulsive Disorder) • Hoarding
Personality Disorders	• Antisocial Disorder (Sociopathy) • BPD (Borderline Personality) • PDP (Dependent Disorder- Inability to be alone with an over-reliance of need from others) • Narcissistic Disorder (Megalomania) • Paranoid Disorder

Psychotic-Schizophrenia	• Schizophrenia
Sleep-Wake Disorders	• Breathing Related Sleep Disorders (Sleep Apnea) • Insomnia • Narcolepsy (Inability to stay awake regardless of circumstances) • Restless Leg Syndrome
Somatic Symptom	• Munchausen Syndrome (Fictitious Disorder-Repeatedly and deliberately acts physical or mental
Substance-Related & Addictive Disorders	• Alcohol-Related Disorders • Cannabis-Related Disorders • Inhalant & Stimulant Use Disorders • Tobacco Use Disorders
Trauma & Stressor Disorders	• Acute Distress (Lasts up to one month) • PTSD (Post Traumatic Stress Disorder) • Reactive Attachment Disorder

Mental illness may not always be present when someone dies by suicide, but it is a contributing factor and exacerbates why an individual thinks suicide is the only answer.

Mental illness increases the risk factors for suicide by affecting your emotions, distorting your thoughts, and changing your behavior.

Living with a mental illness is difficult, and it causes problems for millions around the world. All mental illness requires medical help, not ridicule and judgment. Unfortunately, most times, mentally ill individuals receive neglect, abuse, and discrimination, adding to their guilt and shame.

If we want to act towards reducing suicide rates, then we need to start by breaking the cycle of misinformation and stigma surrounding mental illness.

CHAPTER 9

What They Might Say

Surviving any aspect of suicide is extremely hard. You need to know that being suicidal creates the most dreadful and frightening feelings possible. In addition to attempting to take my own life, I've lived through losing friends and family to suicide. I understand the pain when you are suicidal, and the heartache after surviving a loss. Both cause unbearable pain.

After attempting suicide, I wanted to talk to my family and friends and tell them about what had happened. Fear of judgment kept me from saying anything, and the incident was never discussed. I don't know for certain what your loved one would want to tell you now, but I have a good idea.

This was what I wanted to say, and I believe your loved ones may have as well.

> ➤ I'm sorry. I didn't want to hurt you. I only wanted my horrendous pain to end.

- ➤ You did nothing wrong; don't feel guilty.
- ➤ I was ashamed of my thoughts, so I hid everything.
- ➤ I felt worthless. There was no way anyone could love me.
- ➤ I didn't know how to cope with the pain, sadness, and disappointment that were suffocating me.
- ➤ I didn't want to be a burden to anyone anymore.
- ➤ I did not "choose" to die over living. There was no choice for me.
- ➤ I finally lost all hope and sight of who I was. I couldn't endure the pain anymore.
- ➤ I loved you very much.

Understanding why someone ends their life is challenging, and you may never fully understand why one resorts to suicide. You must know that through their constant torture of pain, fear, and loss of hope, suicide had become their last option to achieve their longing for relief.

CHAPTER 10

What Now?

LET YOURSELF GRIEVE

Now is the time to let yourself grieve. Grief is a natural reaction when losing a loved one. Don't be surprised when you experience emotions like anger, betrayal, rejection, guilt, confusion, denial, loneliness, and pain throughout the grieving process.

All these emotions are part of the process. You need to let yourself go through them and realize it is okay to feel the way you do. The grieving process takes time, and you will move through the process at your own pace.

While going through the grieving process, you will experience emotions that you must deal with rather than ignore. Ignoring your emotions will only make life worse and full of pain.

Denial will be the first emotion you experience. You don't want to think your loved one is gone, or to believe your heart will ever stop hurting. The pain and sorrow in your heart will be excruciating, but restoration is possible.

Once you have accepted you can't bring the individual back, anger will replace the denial. The way you express your anger may differ from that in the past. You may be angry at yourself, but most likely you will be angry at the one you lost. This is normal when you can't do anything to change what happened; you get angry because you have no control.

Your anger may cause you to lash out at whoever is surrounding you. If that consists of family and friends, ensure you talk to them about your anger and what it is really about. Don't leave them wondering what they did wrong.

Sometime along the path of grief, you will feel helpless. You may think about a time you thought you hurt your loved one, thus pushing them to suicide. But the one you lost thought they were causing you pain. There was nothing you did that directly caused their suicidal ideations. Knowing and believing you were not the cause of your loved one's death is crucial to your healing. You must not blame yourself.

Your sadness will increase, possibly causing depression, and you may not feel like getting out of bed. Get up! You must get out of bed so you can work through the grief holding you hostage. You will cry. Let the tears flow and don't stuff them away. To move forward, you need to experience the pain, which is released through tears. Crying does not mean you are weak; it means you care.

Accepting the entire situation will be hard for you. Accepting does not mean forgetting. It doesn't mean you won't be sad ever again. You will probably be sad for the rest of your life, but you will also remember happy moments. As time goes on, the happy memories will outnumber the pain from your loss. The more wonderful memories you experience means you are healing.

Grief hits everyone differently, and the time to work through the sadness and pain varies. You need to grieve for as long as you need to. Don't let anyone tell you it's time to get over it, move on, or to stop thinking about what happened.

You will move on when you are ready, not when someone tells you it's time. Be patient with yourself and realize that you will have good days and bad days dealing with what happened.

The most important way to help yourself move on is to forgive your loved one ... as well as yourself for anything you think you did wrong. Believing the tragedy wasn't your fault will not be easy, but moving in that direction is important for you to start the healing process.

You may have to live with the unanswered question of "Why?" Everyone wants to know why, but the reality is there isn't one answer to ease your mind. Continuing to ask "why" will only prolong your guilt and anger. The only thing you can do is try to understand the pain your loved one experienced.

As you grieve, tap into the help surrounding you; don't push those who love you away. Only you know what support you need to cope with the tragedy. Whether you need friends and family, a spiritual power, or therapy, the worst way to handle your pain is stifling your grief and pretending it didn't happen.

If you are struggling, don't feel embarrassed or hesitate to ask for help. You don't have to go through grief by yourself. You are not alone, and must use the resources you have available to help.

HOW DO YOU MOVE ON?

Experiencing any part of suicide is mortifying. You may not know what to do now, and you are not alone. So, how do you move on?

Honestly, moving on will not be easy; it will depend on you and how long it takes for you to go through the grieving process. Do what helps you heal, not what someone else tells you to do. Don't push the incident out of your mind. If you do, the memories of your loss will haunt you forever.

You need to know the one you lost did not want to hurt you. Instead, they wanted to keep you from the same pain they experienced. Realizing they did not intend to cause you pain is an excellent step towards healing. You must forgive your loved one, regardless of the anger consuming you. Forgiveness has nothing to do with agreeing or accepting the completion of suicide: it is about giving yourself the ability to let the anger and pain go so you can grieve, heal, and move forward.

Don't forget the good times, the smiles, and the laughter. Think about your loved ones often, and don't be afraid to say their name out loud. Talk about the wonderful memories, not what you should have done to help. Focus on remembering who they were, and the wonderful times you spent together. When the tragedy seeps into your thoughts, fill your mind with memories of joy and love, so that the happiness you shared overcomes the sadness.

Stop thinking, "What if," or "If only." The "what ifs" will only make your anguish worse, and eventually unbearable. You do not know if you could have helped, especially if they didn't want help.

You need to believe in your heart the situation was not your fault. Your loved one felt like a burden to everyone, which intensified their pain, leading to more misery.

Losing someone to suicide is not something you will ever get over, and some days you will experience more sadness than others. Take one day at a time and care for yourself instead of beating yourself up over something you couldn't control. Stop asking why; you may never know.

TAKE ACTION

Mental illness and suicide carry negative stigmas that affect thousands of individuals. The responsibility to change the negative effects of the stigma lies with us. You can start making a difference by spreading awareness about mental illness and the role it plays in suicide.

Support suicide prevention and mental illness awareness to increase understanding. These are steps everyone must take to change the epidemic of suicide. The harmful stigma of suicide and mental illness must improve if society wants to stop the increasing suicide rates and help those who are considering suicide.

Instead of shunning or ignoring people with mental illness, be compassionate and non-judgmental. It is important mental illness sufferers know they will receive help instead of ridicule.

Don't avoid the conversation if you suspect someone is struggling. Asking if someone needs help will not make the situation worse, but rather show you care. Always be willing to listen, because it will help individuals move towards getting the help they need.

The most significant factor in changing the viewpoint on mental illness is learning the facts and spreading education about mental illness. Please do not be afraid to talk about suicide or mental illness. Be a part of the change and get involved; you will make a difference.

RESOURCES TO HELP YOU THROUGH YOUR GRIEF:

American Foundation for Suicide Prevention

https://afsp.org/find-support/ive-lost-someone/
resources-loss-survivors/

American Association of Suicidology

http://www.suicidology.org/suicide-survivors/
suicide-loss-survivors

National Suicide Prevention Lifeline

https://suicidepreventionlifeline.org/help-yourself/
loss-survivors/

CHAPTER 11

Do You Have Suicidal Thoughts?

Dealing with suicidal thoughts by yourself is extremely difficult, and not something you should attempt alone. If you are feeling suicidal, reach out to someone, even though you may feel ashamed or afraid. Trust me, I know asking for help is hard, but you need to talk about your thoughts before you act on them.

The ideas going through your head are real, but they are not true. Your situation can change, even if you can't see that now. People around you care, and they will help if you open up and let them know you need it. Even though you feel abandoned and alone, you're not.

When you reach out, it may not feel like anyone understands what you're going through. They may not see the situation from your view, but they see a truth you currently can't.

Call the suicide prevention hotline, go to the emergency room, talk to someone. Please ask for help. Do something besides continuing down a path that leads to destruction or death. Someone will help you.

You have a purpose for being alive. You must believe you are significant, and that your life matters, because everybody matters.

RESOURCES TO HELP YOU
IF YOU ARE HAVING SUICIDAL THOUGHTS:

Suicide Prevention Lifeline
1-800-273-TALK (1-800-273-8255)

https://suicidepreventionlifeline.org/

National Suicide and Crisis Hotline
1-800-SUICIDE (1-800-784-2433)

http://suicidehotlines.com/national.html

National Suicide and Crisis Hotline Speech and
Hearing Impaired
1-800-799-4TTY (1-800-799-4889)

http://suicidehotlines.com/national.html

Closing Thoughts

I was young the first time I thought about suicide. I wanted to drive my car off a bridge: to plunge into the water, sink, and never breathe again. I suffered from mental illness my entire life, but didn't know it until I was in my thirties.

Looking back on my journey, I see how mental illness affected my thoughts and behaviors through the years. Life became a struggle as I got older, and the decisions I made caused a lot of shame and guilt. I didn't notice the depression taking over, or that the emptiness growing in my heart was slowly leading me down a path of destruction.

The suicidal thoughts continued once I experienced the first one. Waking up every day, wanting to die, was the most dreadful feeling I have ever experienced.

I attempted suicide in 2010 when I lost all hope in life. I could no longer endure the unbearable pain and worthlessness I felt; I needed it to stop.

What started as just taking some pain pills to help with my physical pain escalated to never wanting to feel anything again. The hopelessness and emptiness never ended, no matter what I did. I didn't want to prolong my suffering, and my want turned to a burning desire, which led to action.

That night, my mind was empty of all thoughts except one: *dying.* I couldn't stop the horrible, toxic thoughts that attacked me. The distorted thoughts whirling in my mind held no truth, but I couldn't see anything positive to help change my views.

There were no thoughts about loved ones or how they would be affected by my actions. I already knew what I was doing was best for everyone. Once I started down the destructive path on my way to suicide, I lost control; I couldn't stop until the pain ended. The accumulation of pain, misery, hopelessness, and feelings of worthlessness finally pushed me to suicide.

I endured that never-ending pain, and knowing I had no way out terrified me. My fear of living another day in constant pain led me to believe I had no purpose. I no longer knew who I was or why I even existed. My hope disappeared, and staying alive wasn't an option. I wasn't trying to hurt anyone except myself.

I wish I would have felt safe asking for help before I had gotten to the point of suicide. I believe if I had received help, that night never would have happened.

I am not trying to tell you how you should feel about suicide. I want to help you understand how a person turns to suicide and why they act upon those thoughts. I am sharing my suicide experience with you to show you what one goes through when acting on suicidal thoughts. Not when it's a passing thought, but when you are active and in the moment. A time when all feelings, desires, and actions become distorted and uncontrollable.

I can't truly explain the way I felt that night. I wish I could describe my despair, because I don't believe anyone can completely understand the feeling unless they experience it.

I know what it feels like to lose all hope, and when it's gone, there is nothing left inside your soul to encourage you to keep your hold on life. Hope truly is the anchor for your soul: it keeps you looking forward to waking up every day and wanting to live.

Hebrews 6:19 *"This hope is a strong and trustworthy anchor for our souls. It leads us through the curtain into God's inner sanctuary."* [22]

Source Notes

1. NAMI: National Alliance on Mental Illness. "Mental Health by the Numbers," last updated March 2021. https://www.nami.org/mhstats.

2. Galvin, Gaby. "The U.S. Suicide Rate Has Soared Since 1999," U.S. News, accessed October 8, 2021. https://www.usnews.com/news/healthiest-communities/articles/2020-04-08/cdc-report-suicide-rate-up-35-since-1999%E2%80%A9.

3. Pratt, Kim. "What are Cognitive Distortions," Healthy Psych, accessed August 6, 2019. https://healthypsych.com/psychology-tools-what-are-cognitive-distortions/.

4. Dictionary.com. "'Deformed' definition," accessed October 6, 2021. https://www.dictionary.com/browse/deformed.

5. Futch, Richelle. "A Lesson in Mindfulness: The 3 States of Mind," Solution Focused Parenting, accessed June 9, 2020. https://www.solutionfocusedparenting.com/a-lesson-in-mindfulness-the-3-states-of-mind/.

6. Valley Behavioral Health System. "Understanding Suicidal Ideation," Valley Behavioral, accessed January 26, 2018. https://www.valleybehavioral.com/ suicidal-ideation/signs-symptoms-causes/.

7. Ricee, Susanne. "Subconscious vs. Unconscious: The Complete Comparison," Diversity for Social Impact, accessed October 6, 2021. https://diversity.social/ unconscious-vs-subconscious/

8. Wikipedia. "Freedom of Choice," accessed October 22, 2019. https://en.wikipedia.org/wiki/Freedom_of_choice.

9. Rational Wiki. "False Dilemma," accessed October 22, 2019. https://rationalwiki.org/wiki/False_dilemma

10. Heckler, Richard A. "The Suicidal Trance," Alliance of Hope, accessed August 6, 2019. https://allianceofhope. org/richard-heckler-on-the-suicidal-trance/.

11. American Psychiatric Association. "What is DSM and Why is it Important," accessed June 7, 2021. https:// www.psychiatry.org/psychiatrists/practice/dsm/ feedback-and-questions/frequently-asked-questions.

12. American Psychiatric Association: "Diagnostic and Statistical Manual of Mental Disorders, Fifth Edition. Arlington, VA, American Psychiatric Association, 2013.

13. Soba NJ. "What's the Difference Between Mental Illness and Mental Disorder," Soba New Jersey, accessed March 3, 2021. https://sobanewjersey.com/ blog/whats-the-difference-between-mental-ill- ness-and-mental-disorder/.

14. CDC Centers for Disease Control and Prevention. "Cognitive Impairment: A Call for Action, Now!" accessed July 25, 2021. https://www.cdc.gov/aging/pdf/cognitive_impairment/cogimp_poilicy_final.pdf

15. Baton Rouge Behavioral Hospital. "The Surprising History of Mental Illness Treatment," accessed June 2, 2021. https://batonrougebehavioral.com/the-surprising-history-of-mental-illness-treatment/ATON ROUGE BEHAVIORAL HOSPITAL

16. Open Library Press Books. "History of Mental Illness," accessed June 2, 2021. https://ecampusontario.pressbooks.pub/testbookje/chapter/history-of-mental-illness/.

17. Editorial Staff. "The History & Evolution of Mental Health & Treatment." American Addiction Centers, Sunrise House Treatment Center, last updated August 5, 2020. https://sunrisehouse.com/research/history-evolution-mental-health-treatment/.

18. Historic England. "From Bethlehem to Bedlam—England's First Mental Institution," accessed June 22, 2021. https://historicengland.org.uk/research/inclusive-heritage/disability-history/1050-1485/from-bethlehem-to-bedlam/.

19. Agape Treatment Center. "How Mental Health Conditions Can Increase Suicide Risks," accessed June 16, 2021. https://www.agapetc.com/mental-health-and-suicide/.

20. Mental Health First Aid USA. "5 Surprising Mental Health Statistics," accessed June 3, 2021. https://www.mentalhealthfirstaid. org/2019/02/5-surprising-mental-health-statistics/.

21. Cherry, Kendra. "A List of Psychological Disorders," Verywell Mind, last updated on March 19, 2020. https://www.verywellmind. com/a-list-of-psychological-disorders-2794776.

22. NLT Bible. "Hebrews Chapter 6 Verse 19, This hope is a strong and trustworthy anchor," accessed August 11, 2021. https://www.bible.com/bible/116/HEB.6.19.nlt.

MENTAL DISORDER ILLNESS DEFINITION REFERENCES—RELATED TO NOTE NUMBER (21)

1. Bhandari, Smitha, MD. "Dissociative Identity Disorder (Multiple Personality Disorder)," WebMD, last modified January 22, 2020. https://www.webmd.com/ mental-health/dissociative-identity-disorder-multiple-personality-disorder#4.

2. Bhandari, Smitha, MD. "Intellectual Disability," Grow by WebMD, last reviewed September 12, 2020. https://www.webmd.com/parenting/baby/ intellectual-disability-mental-retardation#1.

3. Bhandari, Smitha, MD. "Munchausen Syndrome," WebMD, accessed July 2, 2020. https://www.webmd. com/mental-health/munchausen-syndrome#1.

4. Casarella, Jennifer, MD. "Mental Health and Dissociative Amnesia," WebMD, last reviewed April 21, 2021. https://www.webmd.com/mental-health/dissociative-amnesia#1.

5. Mayo Clinic. "Body Dysmorphic Disorder," accessed July 2, 2020. https://www.mayoclinic.org/diseases-conditions/body-dysmorphic-disorder/symptoms-causes/syc-20353938.

6. Mayo Clinic. "Intermittent Explosive Disorder," accessed July 2, 2020. https://www.mayoclinic.org/diseases-conditions/intermittent-explosive-disorder/symptoms-causes/syc-20373921#:~:text=Overview,of%20proportion%20to%20the%20situation.

7. Mayo Clinic. "Kleptomania," accessed July 2, 2020. https://www.mayoclinic.org/diseases-conditions/kleptomania/symptoms-causes/syc-20364732.

8. Mayo Clinic. "Narcolepsy," accessed July 2, 2020. https://www.mayoclinic.org/diseases-conditions/narcolepsy/symptoms-causes/syc-20375497.

9. Morin, Amy. "Pyromania Causes and Treatment," Verywell Mind, accessed July 2, 2020. https://www.verywellmind.com/what-is-a-pyromaniac-4160050.

10. Psychology Today. "Dependent Personality Disorder," last modified 2019. https://www.psychologytoday.com/us/conditions/dependent-personality-disorder.

Author Summary

Bobbie is an advocate for increasing mental illness and suicide awareness in today's society. Having struggled with suicide herself, Bobbie has a profound understanding of the pain involved in this devastating event, from all perspectives. In her book, Bobbie shares her first-hand experience and direct knowledge to help the reader understand the motivations behind suicide and providing avenues for post-traumatic healing. Bobbie strongly believes that spreading information about suicide will help diffuse the current stigma surrounding this controversial topic.

Bobbie grew up in St. Maries, Idaho and currently lives in sunny California.